MW00978664

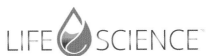

Copyright © 2017
Life Science Publishing
1.800.336.6308
www.DiscoverLSP.com

Printed in the United States of America
10 9 8 7 6 5 4 3 2 1

Life Science Publishing is the publisher of this book and is not responsible for its content. The information contained herein is for educational purposes only and as a guideline for your personal use. It should not be used as a substitute for medical counseling with a health professional. Neither the author nor publisher accepts responsibility for such use.

The essential oils and supplemental products discussed at length in this book are the sole product of Young Living Essential Oils. The authors and publisher are completely separate entities from Young Living Essential Oils. Products mentioned may be reformulated, discontinued, expanded, or enhanced by Young Living Essential Oils at any given time.

Neither the authors nor the publisher advocate the use of any other essential oils without the Seed to Seal guarantee. Even minor changes in the quality of an essential oil may render it, at best, useless and, at worst, dangerous. The use of essential oils should be done with thorough study, watchful care, and judicious prudence.

INTRODUCTION

This booklet contains over 50 recipes to provide new and seasoned members with fun easy recipes to create and use during each of the four seasons.

There are recipes for roll-ons, sprays, scrubs, bath salts, drinks, and more. We hope to inspire people to use their starter kit essential oils and explore additional essential oils too. These recipes are great to use for Make & Take events for all of the seasons.

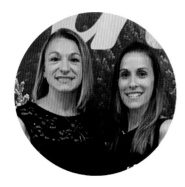

Oily Yours,

Chelsa Bruno & Dana Ripepe

Disclaimer: This booklet is for educational purposes only. We do not diagnose, treat, cure, or prevent any disease. If you are suffering from any disease, illness, or injury it is your responsibility to consult with your Physician.

The publisher and authors can not be held liable for the results you experience from the use of any of these recipes. For those with sensitive skin, it is recommended to test each recipe on a small area of your skin before using on larger areas.

TABLE OF CONTENTS
WINTER TIME RECIPES

Cozy By The Fire Room Spray 2

PanAway Rosemary Bath Salts 2

Holiday Spirit Diffuser Blend 4

Peppermint Delight Room Spray 5

Joyful Sugar Scrub 7

Holiday Cheer Body Spray 7

Diffuser Ornaments...8

Peppermint Hot Chocolate 10

Hot Orange Spice Drink 10

Romance is in the Air Diffuser Blend 12

Light Your Fire Body Scrub 13

Happy Lady Body Spray 14

Romantic Bath Salts 14

Sensual Couples Massage...17

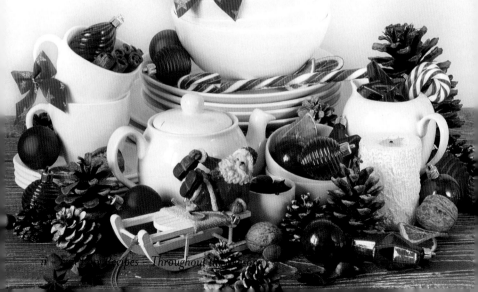

SPRING TIME RECIPES

Spring Breeze Room Spray...20
Floral Perfume Roll-On 20
Spring Bloom Diffuser Blend...22
Spring is in the Air Roll-On..22
Citrus Sugar Scrub...24
Breeze of Happiness Diffuser Blend...........................24
Lemongrass Body Wash 26
Orange Cream Body Scrub 27
Ultimate Happy Camper Spray 28
Happy Pets Spray...28
Seasonal Wellness Support Capsule 30
Thieves Tile/Tub Cleaner...32
Stainless Steel Cleaner 32
Citrus Start Smoothie...34
Pomegranate Orange Punch 35

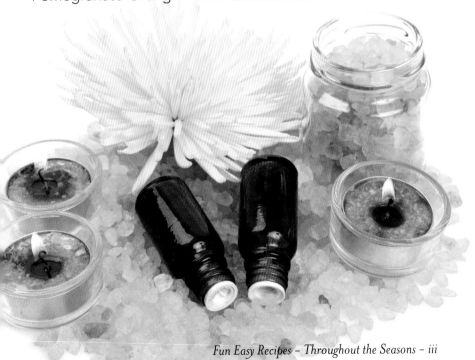

SUMMER TIME RECIPES

Summer Relaxation Body Scrub...................................38

Ocean Mist Air Freshener...38

Citrus Loving Diffuser Blend..40

Vacation Time Bath Salts 40

Grapefruit Lime Sugar Scrub.......................................42

Summer Time Body Spray..42

Summer Bliss Diffuser Blend 44

Cooling Roll-On...44

Soothing Skin Cream 46

After Swimming Roll-On...47

Strawberry Lemonade..48

Frozen Berry Lime Margarita 49

AUTUMN TIME RECIPES

Autumn Breeze Roll-On 52

Sugar & Spice Room Spray 52

Autumn Time Sugar Scrub 54

Yummy Apple Pie Diffuser Blend 54

Pumpkin Spice Foaming Hand Soap 56

Fall Delight Foot Soak 56

Autumn Spice Diffuser Blend 58

School Days Immune System Support 58

Healthy School Time Hair 61

Homework Time Roll-On 61

Dreamy Chocolate Smoothie 62

Hot Cinnamon Spice Drink 62

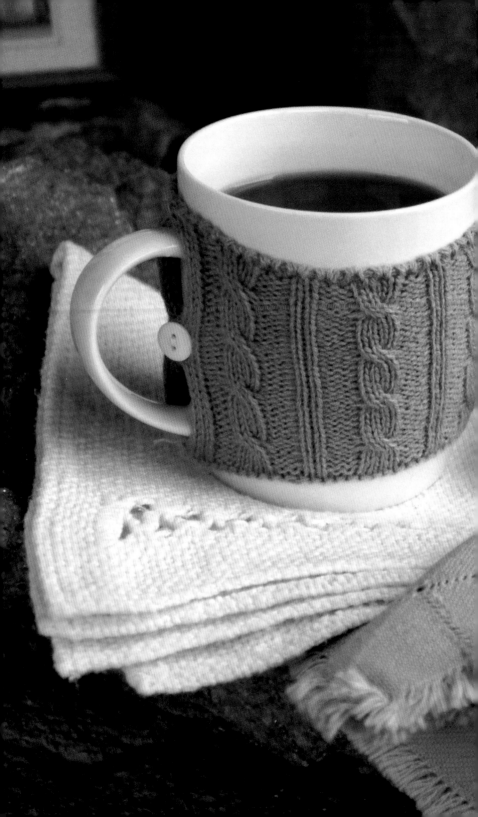

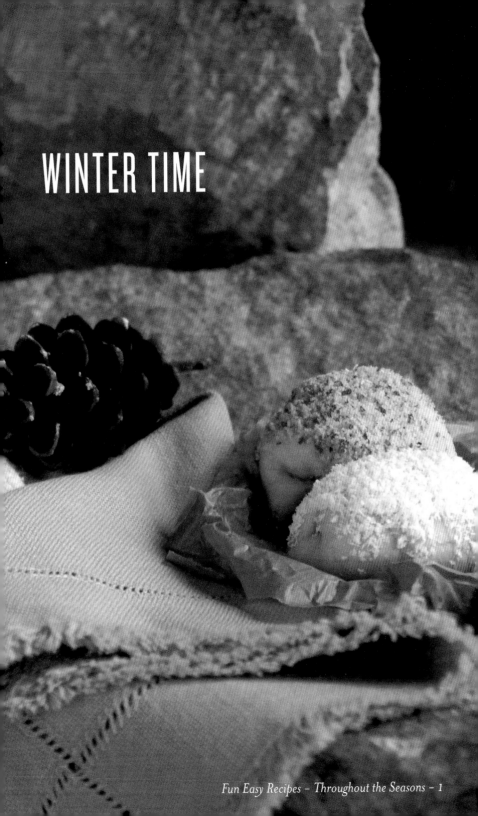

WINTER TIME

Cozy by the Fire Room Spray

Ingredients:
- 5 drops Cinnamon Bark Essential Oil
- 5 drops Orange Essential Oil
- 5 drops Clove Essential Oil
- Water
- 2 oz Glass Spray Bottle

Directions:
1. Add the Essential Oils into the spray bottle
2. Fill with water and put on the spray bottle top
3. Shake well before spraying into the air to create a cozy, calming atmosphere

PanAway Rosemary Bath Salts

Ingredients:
- 5 drops PanAway Essential Oil
- 3 drops Rosemary Essential Oil
- 1/3 cup Epsom Salt
- 4 oz Glass Mason Jar

Directions:
1. Put the Epsom Salt, PanAway and Rosemary Essential Oils into a glass bowl
2. Mix the ingredients together and place the mixture into the jar
3. Add 1 tablespoon of the mixture into your bath water for muscle and joint support

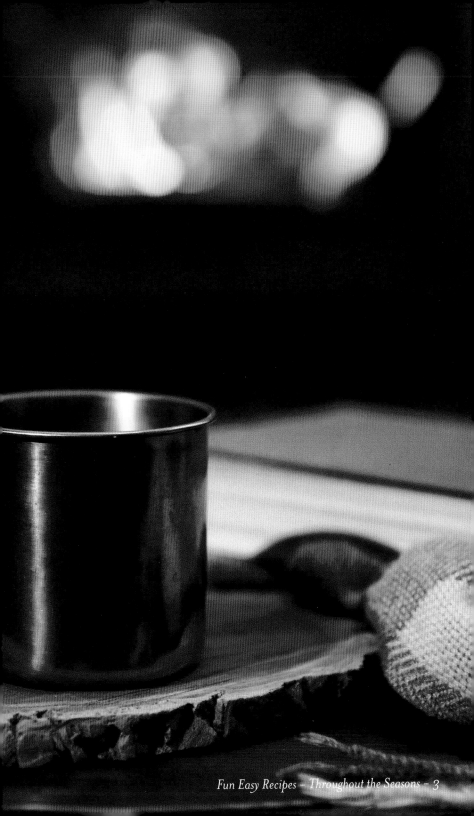

Holiday Spirit Diffuser Blend

Ingredients:
- 3 drops Christmas Spirit Essential Oil
- 2 drops Joy Essential Oil
- Water
- Diffuser

Directions:
1. Add water to the fill line of the diffuser
2. Put Christmas Spirit and Joy Essential Oils into the water
3. Put the top of the diffuser on and press the on button
4. Breathe in some Holiday Spirit

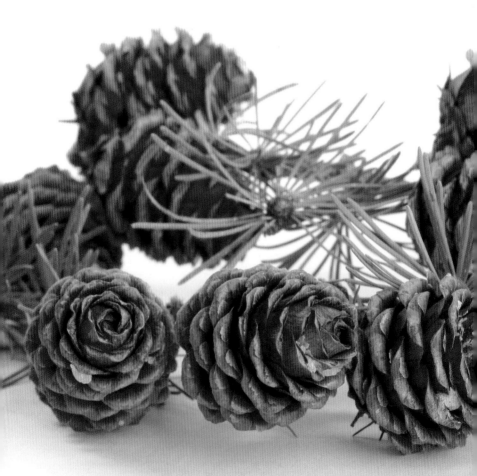

Peppermint Delight Room Spray

<u>Ingredients:</u>
- 6 drops Peppermint Essential Oil
- 3 drops Ylang Ylang Essential Oil
- Water
- 2 oz Glass Spray Bottle

<u>Directions:</u>
1. Add Peppermint and Ylang Ylang Essential Oils into the spray bottle and fill with water. Put on the spray bottle top.
2. Shake well before spraying into the air

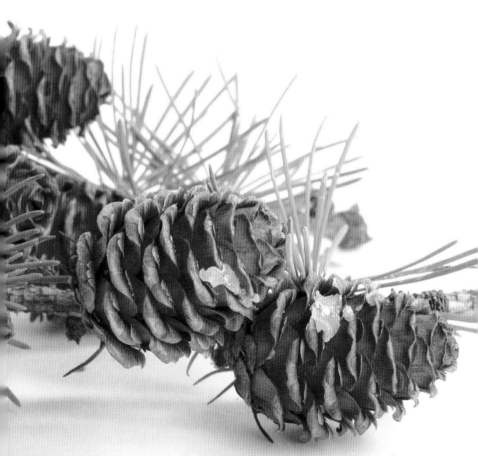

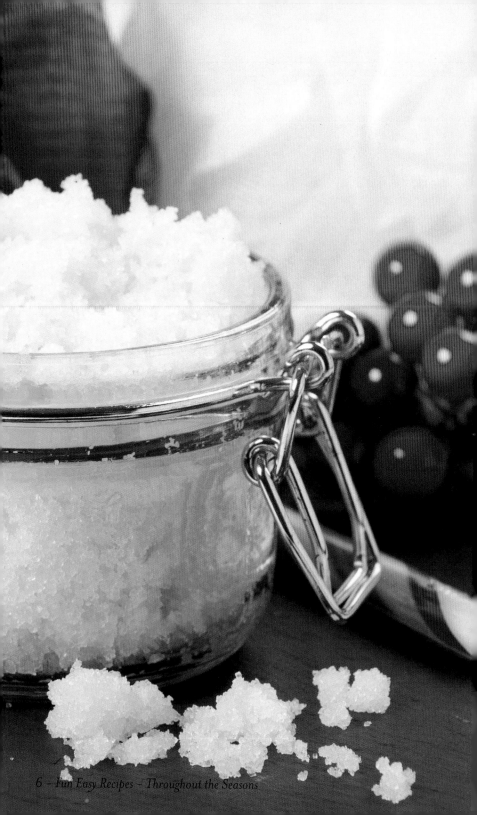

Joyful Sugar Scrub

Ingredients:
- 4 drops Joy Essential Oil
- 3 drops Peppermint Essential Oil
- ½ cup Raw Sugar
- ¼ cup Virgin Coconut Oil
- 4 oz Glass Mason Jar

Directions:
1. Put the Raw Sugar, Coconut Oil, Joy and Peppermint Essential Oils into a glass bowl
2. Mix the ingredients together
3. Place the mixture into the jar
4. Use this invigorating scrub to exfoliate your body

Holiday Cheer Body Spray

Ingredients:
- 6 drops Stress Away Essential Oil
- 4 drops Christmas Spirit Essential Oil
- Water
- 2 oz Glass Spray Bottle

Directions:
1. Add the Essential Oils into the spray bottle
2. Fill with water and put on the spray bottle top
3. Shake well before spraying onto your body

Diffuser Ornaments

Ingredients:
- Oven-Bake Clay
- Holiday Stamps
- Ornament Shaped Cookie Cutter
- Wooden Stick

Directions:
1. Use a rolling pin to flatten the clay
2. Cut out ornament shape in the clay using the cookie cutter
3. Use the wooden stick to make a hole at the top to be able to add string after its cooked
4. Decorate the ornament with the holiday stamps
5. Put parchment paper on a baking sheet
6. Place the ornaments on the parchment paper and bake at 275°F for 12 minutes
7. Let it cool and then add string to the ornaments
8. Hang ornaments
9. Add 1 drop of your favorite Young Living Essential Oil to the ornaments

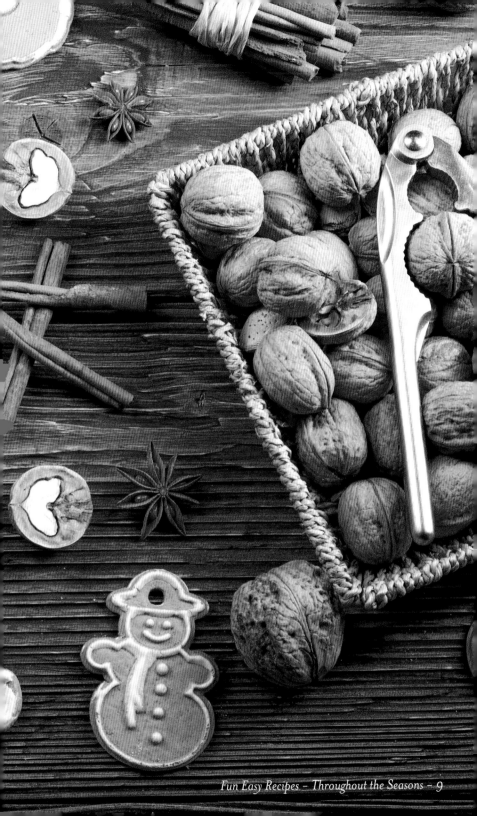

Peppermint Hot Chocolate

Ingredients:
- 1 drop Peppermint Vitality Essential Oil
- 2 Tbsp Unsweetened Cocoa Powder
- 1 Tbsp Raw Honey
- 1 cup Milk (dairy or non-dairy)

Directions:
1. Over medium heat, stir the milk in a saucepan until hot (not boiling)
2. Pour the milk into a mug and add the cocoa powder, raw honey and Peppermint Vitality Essential Oil
3. Stir well and enjoy

Hot Orange Spice Drink

Ingredients:
- 1 drop Clove Vitality Essential Oil
- 1 drop Cinnamon Bark Vitality Essential Oil
- 1 cup Orange Juice
- 1 Tbsp Raw Honey
- $1/8$ cup Water

Directions:
1. Combine the orange juice and water in a saucepan
2. Over medium heat, stir until hot (not boiling)
3. Pour into a mug and add the honey and essential oils
4. Stir well and enjoy

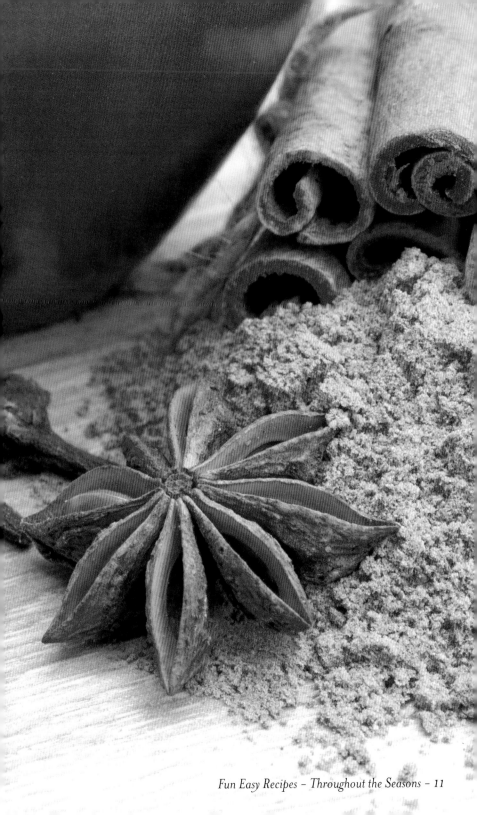

Ingredients:
- 2 drops Joy Essential Oil
- 1 drop Bergamot Essential Oil
- 1 drop Cedarwood Essential Oil
- 1 drop Lavender Essential Oil
- Water
- Diffuser

Directions:
1. Add water to the fill line of the diffuser
2. Put Joy, Bergamot, Cedarwood and Lavender Essential Oils into the water
3. Put the top of the diffuser on and press the on button
4. Enjoy the romantic atmosphere

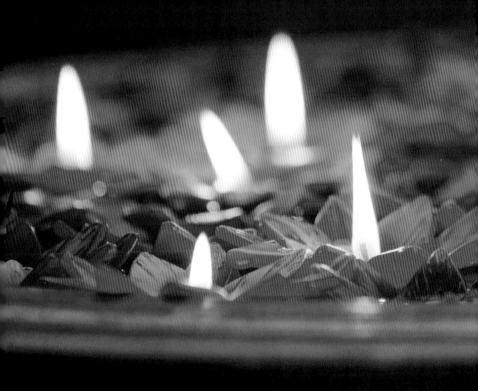

Light Your Fire Body Scrub

Ingredients:
- 4 drops Ylang Ylang Essential Oil
- 3 drops Black Spruce Essential Oil
- ½ cup Raw Sugar
- ¼ cup Virgin Coconut Oil
- 4 oz Glass Mason Jar

Directions:
1. Put the Raw Sugar, Coconut Oil, Ylang Ylang and Black Spruce Essential Oils into a glass bowl
2. Mix the ingredients together
3. Place the mixture into the jar
4. Use this scrub to uplift and exfoliate your body

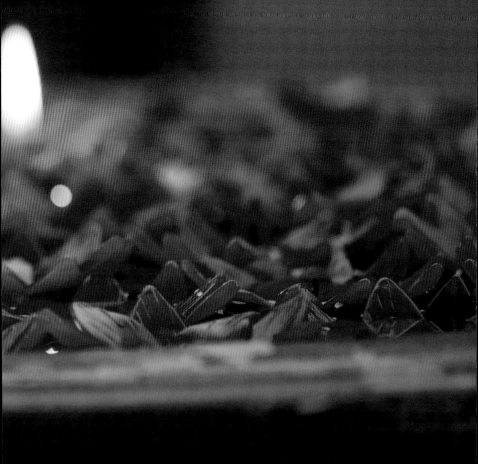

Happy Lady Body Spray

Ingredients:
- 8 drops Live with Passion Essential Oil
- 8 drops Sensation Essential Oil
- Water
- 2 oz Glass Spray Bottle

Directions:
1. Add the Essential Oils into the spray bottle
2. Fill with water and put on the spray bottle top
3. Shake well before spraying onto your body

Romantic Bath Salts

Ingredients:
- 4 drops Ylang Ylang Essential Oil
- 3 drops Idaho Blue Spruce Essential Oil
- 1/3 cup Epsom Salt
- 4 oz Glass Mason Jar

Directions:
1. Put the Epsom Salt, Ylang Ylang and Idaho Blue Spruce
   Essential Oils into a glass bowl
2. Mix the ingredients together and
   place the mixture into the jar
3. Add 1 tablespoon of the mixture
   into your bath water for relaxation

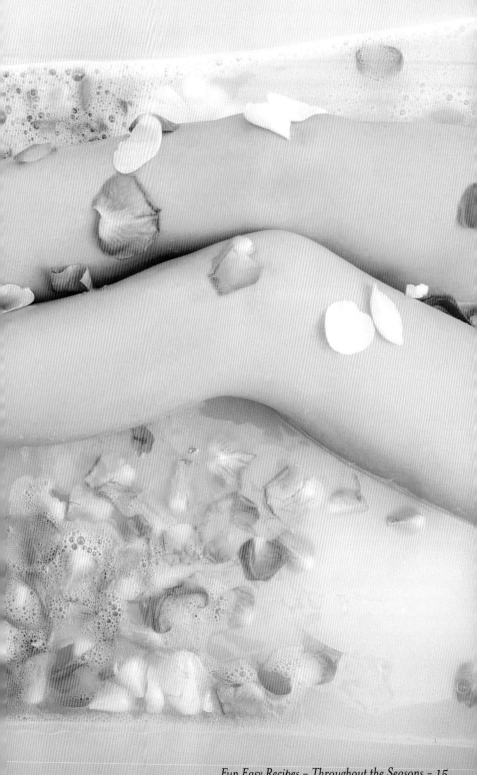

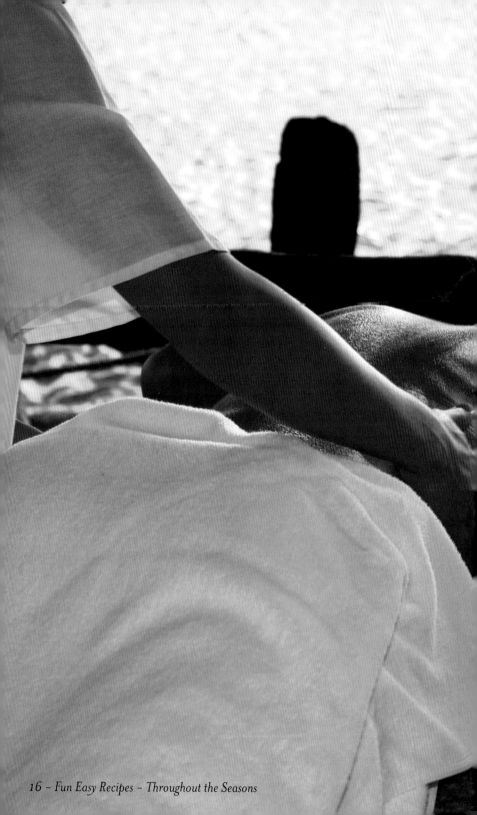

Sensual Couples Massage

Ingredients:
- 10 drops Ylang Ylang Essential Oil
- 5 drops Sandalwood Essential Oil
- 5 drops Orange Essential Oil
- Sensation Massage Oil / V-6 Vegetable Oil
- 4 oz Glass Pump Bottle

Directions:
1. Add the Essential Oils into the glass pump bottle
2. Fill with Sensation Massage Oil and put on the bottle top
3. Shake well before applying to the body for a relaxing massage

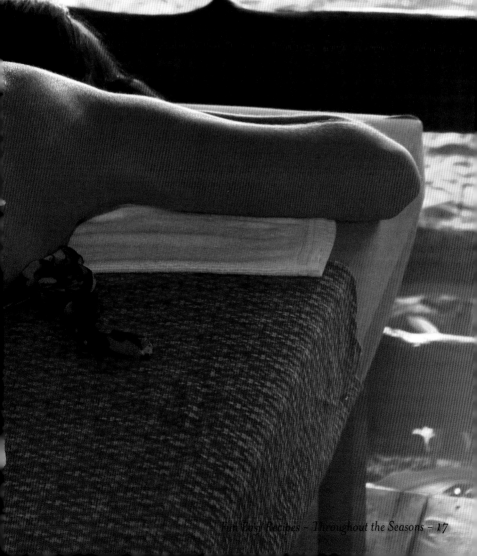

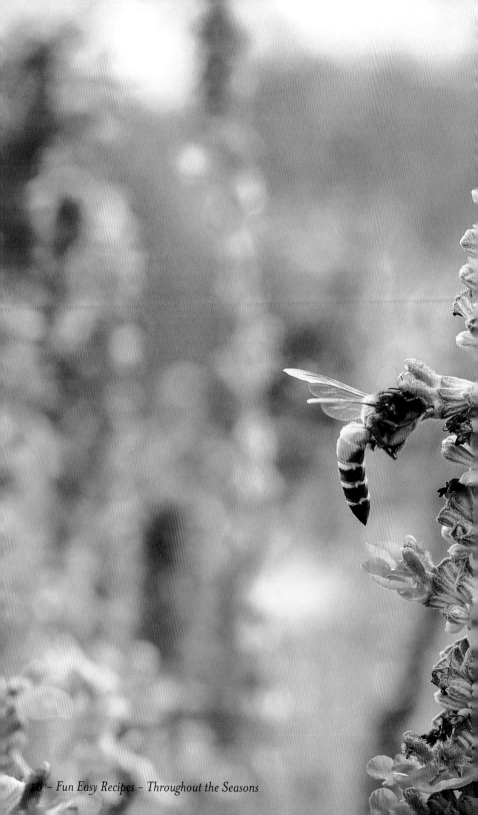

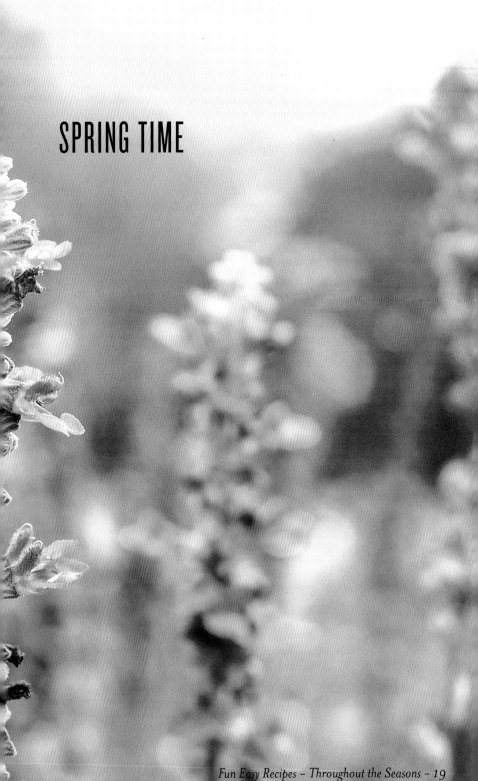

SPRING TIME

Spring Breeze Room Spray

Ingredients:
- 8 drops Joy Essential Oil
- 8 drops Ylang Ylang Essential Oil
- Water
- 2 oz Glass Spray Bottle

Directions:
1. Add the Essential Oils into the spray bottle
2. Fill with water and put on the spray bottle top
3. Shake well before spraying into the air

Floral Perfume Roll-On

Ingredients:
- 6 drops Geranium Essential Oil
- 6 drops Bergamot Essential Oil
- 6 drops Joy Essential Oil
- V-6 Vegetable Oil (or Liquid Coconut Oil)
- 10 mL Glass Roll-On Bottle

Directions:
1. Add the Essential Oils into the roll-on bottle
2. Fill with V-6 Vegetable Oil and put on the roll-on top
3. Apply onto your wrists and chest

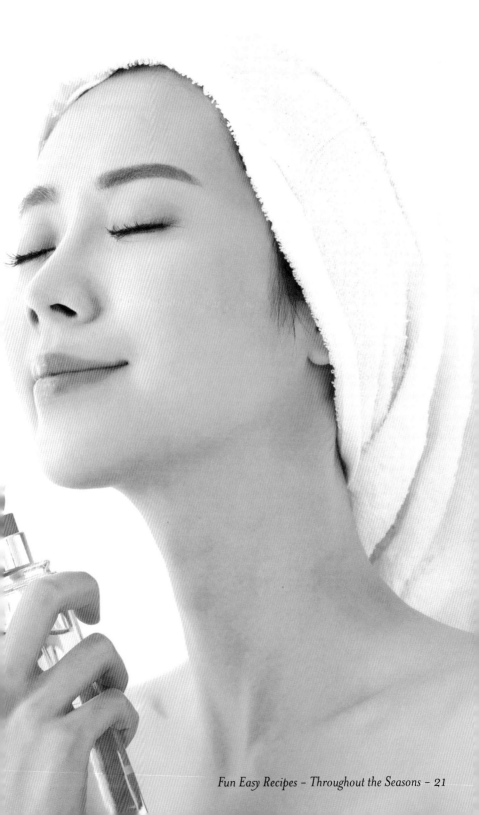

Spring Bloom Diffuser Blend

Ingredients:
- 2 drops Lavender Essential Oil
- 2 drops Peppermint Essential Oil
- 2 drops R.C. Essential Oil
- Water
- Diffuser

Directions:
1. Add water to the fill line of the diffuser
2. Put Lavender, Peppermint and R.C. Essential Oils into the water
3. Put the top of the diffuser on and press the on button
4. Breathe in the happy scents of Spring

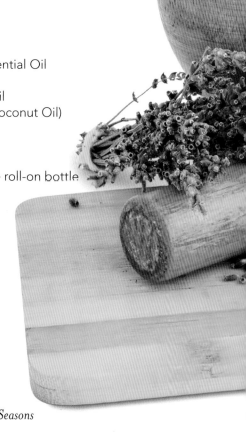

Spring is in the Air Roll-On

Ingredients:
- 6 drops Peace & Calming Essential Oil
- 6 drops Lemon Essential Oil
- 6 drops Geranium Essential Oil
- V-6 Vegetable Oil (or Liquid Coconut Oil)
- 10 mL Glass Roll-On Bottle

Directions:
1. Add the Essential Oils into the roll-on bottle
2. Fill with V-6 Vegetable Oil and put on the roll-on top
3. Apply onto your wrists and behind your ears

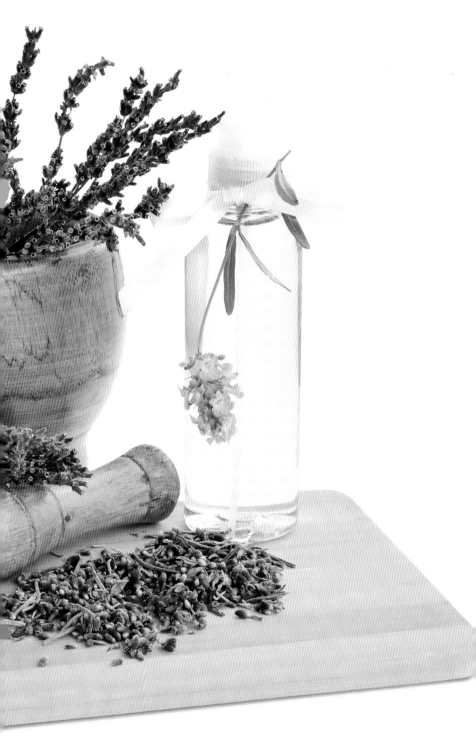

Citrus Sugar Scrub

Ingredients:
- 5 drops Citrus Fresh Essential Oil
- ½ cup Raw Sugar
- ¼ cup Virgin Coconut Oil
- 4 oz Glass Mason Jar

Directions:
1. Put the Raw Sugar, Coconut Oil and Citrus Fresh Essential Oil into a glass bowl
2. Mix the ingredients together
3. Place the mixture into the jar
4. Use this scrub to exfoliate your hands or body

Breeze of Happiness Diffuser Blend

Ingredients:
- 2 drops Joy Essential Oil
- 2 drops Stress Away Essential Oil
- 2 drops Lavender Essential Oil
- Water
- Diffuser

Directions:
1. Add water to the fill line of the diffuser
2. Put Joy, Stress Away and Lavender Essential Oils into the water
3. Put the top of the diffuser on and press the on button
4. Breathe in the happy scents of Spring

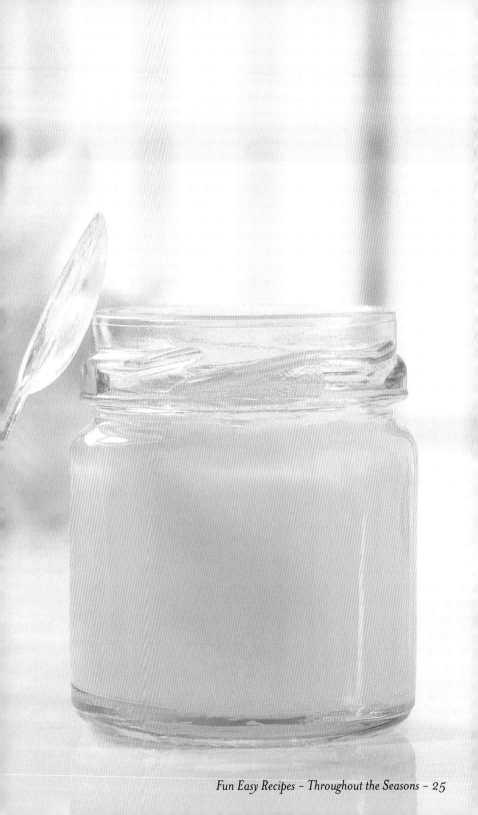

Lemongrass Body Wash

Ingredients:
- 10 drops Lemongrass Essential Oil
- 3 Tbsp Castile Soap
- Water
- 8 ½ oz Glass Foaming Bottle

Directions:
1. Add Lemongrass Essential Oil into the foaming bottle
2. Add Castile Soap and fill the bottle with water
3. Put on the foaming bottle top
4. Use this to cleanse your body and support the circulatory system

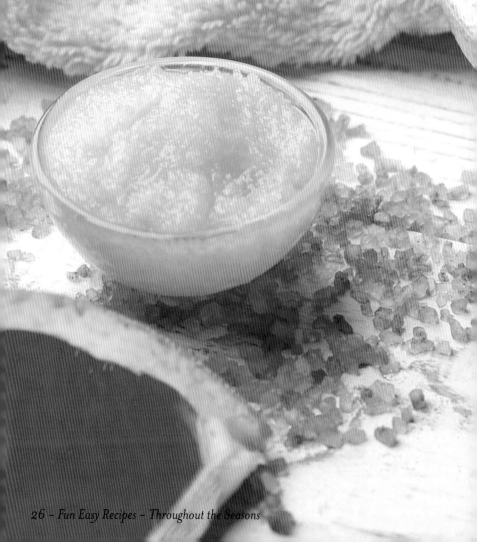

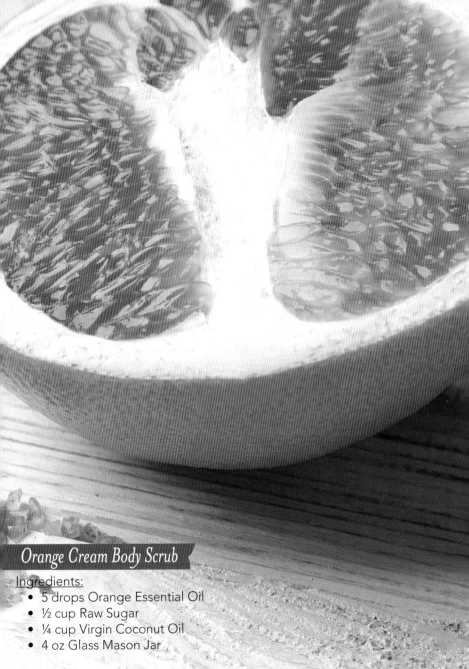

Orange Cream Body Scrub

Ingredients:
- 5 drops Orange Essential Oil
- ½ cup Raw Sugar
- ¼ cup Virgin Coconut Oil
- 4 oz Glass Mason Jar

Directions:
1. Put the Raw Sugar, Coconut Oil and Orange Essential Oil into a glass bowl
2. Mix the ingredients together
3. Place the mixture into the jar
4. Use this scrub to exfoliate your body

Ultimate Happy Camper Spray

Ingredients:
- 10 drops Purification Essential Oil
- 10 drops Eucalyptus Radiata Essential Oil
- 10 drops Lavender Essential Oil
- 10 drops Peppermint Essential Oil
- 10 drops Geranium Essential Oil
- Water
- 2 oz Glass Spray Bottle

Directions:
1. Add the Essential Oils into the spray bottle and fill with water. Then put on the spray bottle top.
2. Shake well before using.
   Spray onto your body when outside.

Happy Pets Spray

Ingredients:
- 5 drops Peppermint Essential Oil
- 5 drops Tea Tree Essential Oil
- 5 drops Rosemary Essential Oil
- Water
- 2 oz Glass Spray Bottle

Directions:
1. Add the Essential Oils into the spray bottle and fill with water. Then put on the spray bottle top.
2. Shake well before using.
   Spray onto your pet when outside.

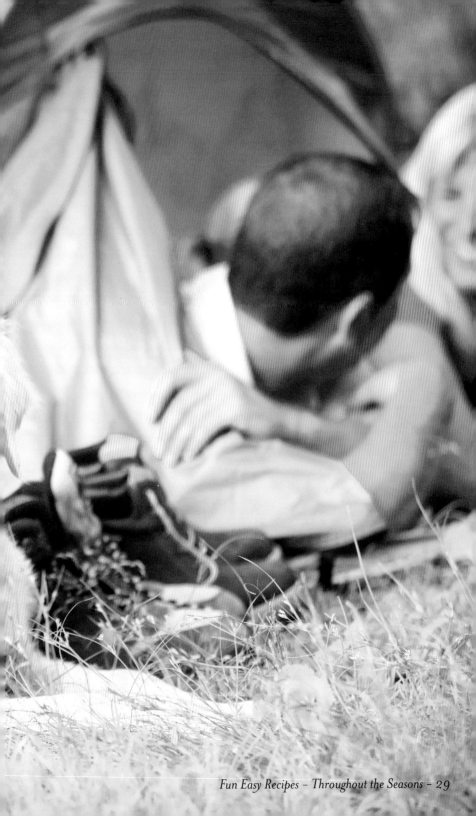

Seasonal Wellness Support Capsule

Ingredients:
- 6 drops Lavender Vitality Essential Oil
- 4 drops Copaiba Vitality Essential Oil
- Vegetable Capsules

Directions:
1. Add the Essential Oils into the capsule
2. Ingest one capsule daily for
   Seasonal Wellness Support

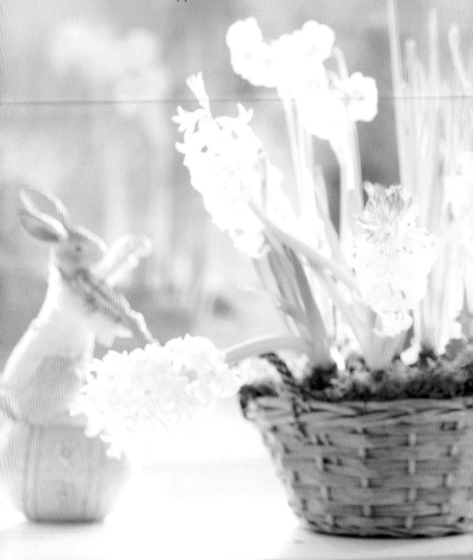

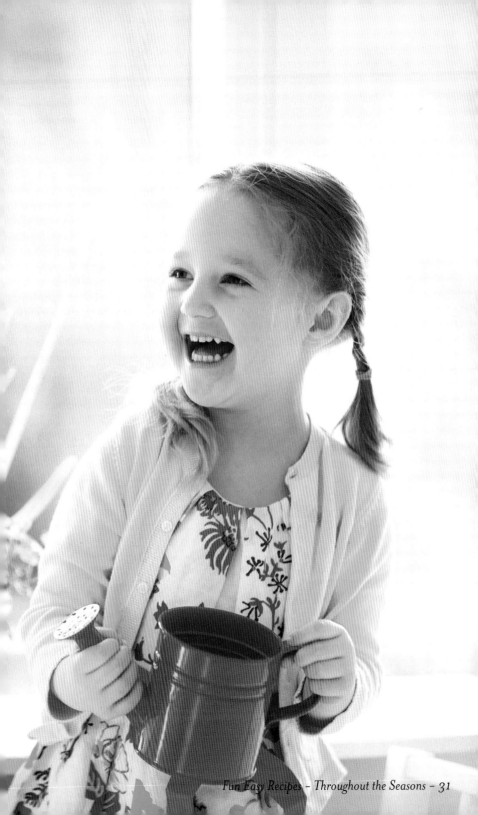

Thieves Tile/Tub Cleaner

Ingredients:
- 2 capfuls Thieves Household Cleaner
- ½ cup Baking Soda
- 2 Tbsp Water

Directions:
1. Put the Thieves Household Cleaner, Baking Soda and Water into a glass bowl
2. Mix the ingredients together
3. Place some of the mixture onto a sponge to clean tiles and bathtub

Stainless Steel Cleaner

Ingredients:
- 1 capful Thieves Household Cleaner
- ¼ cup Liquid Coconut Oil
- Water
- 7 oz Glass/Aluminum Spray Bottle

Directions:
1. Put the Thieves Household Cleaner and Coconut Oil into the spray bottle
2. Fill with water and shake well before using

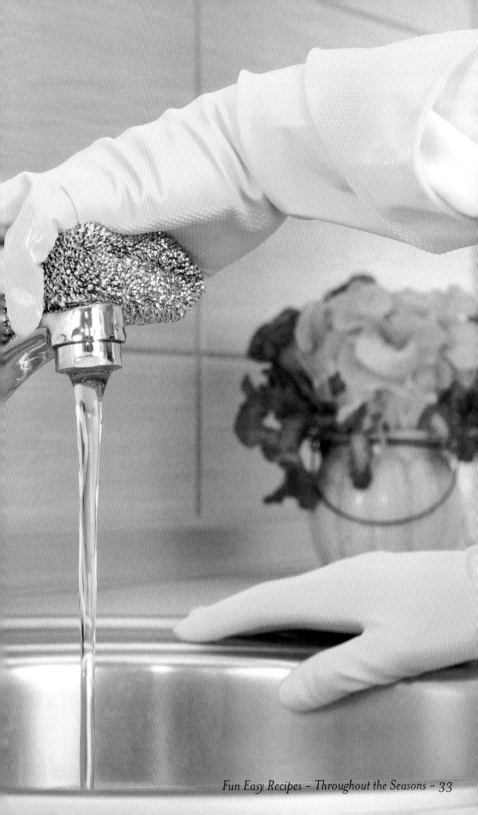

Citrus Start Smoothie

Ingredients:

- 5 oz Pineapple Juice
- 3 oz NingXia Red
- 1 cup Ice
- 1 cup frozen Peaches
- ½ cup fresh Raspberries

Directions:

1. Pour the Pineapple Juice, NingXia Red and ice into a blender
2. Add the Peaches and Raspberries into the blender
3. Blend, then pour into a glass, drink, and enjoy

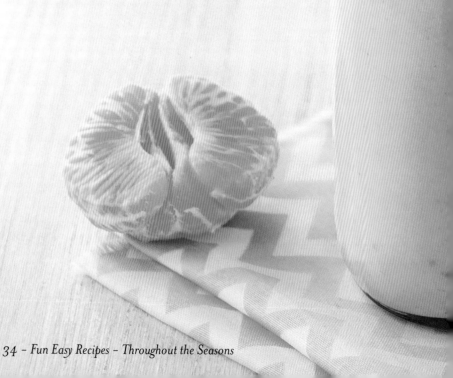

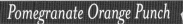
Pomegranate Orange Punch

Ingredients:
- 5 drops Orange Vitality Essential Oil
- 3 oz NingXia Red
- 1 cup Pomegranate Juice
- 1 Liter Bottle Seltzer
- 1 cup Water
- 2 Tbsp Raw Sugar
- 2 peeled & diced Oranges
- 1 cup diced fresh Pineapple

Directions:
1. Pour all of the ingredients into a glass pitcher and mix together
2. Place in refrigerator for an hour before serving
3. Drink and enjoy

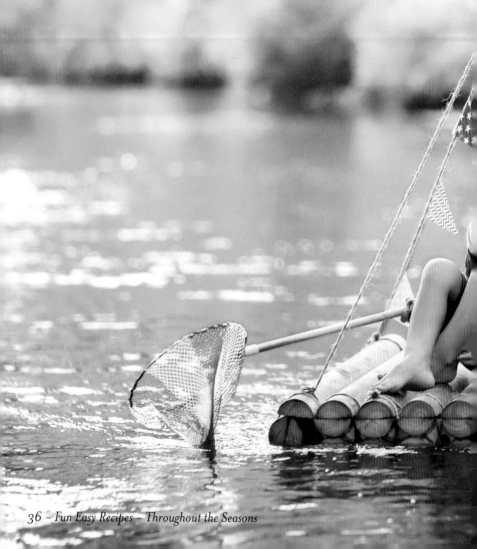

SUMMER TIME

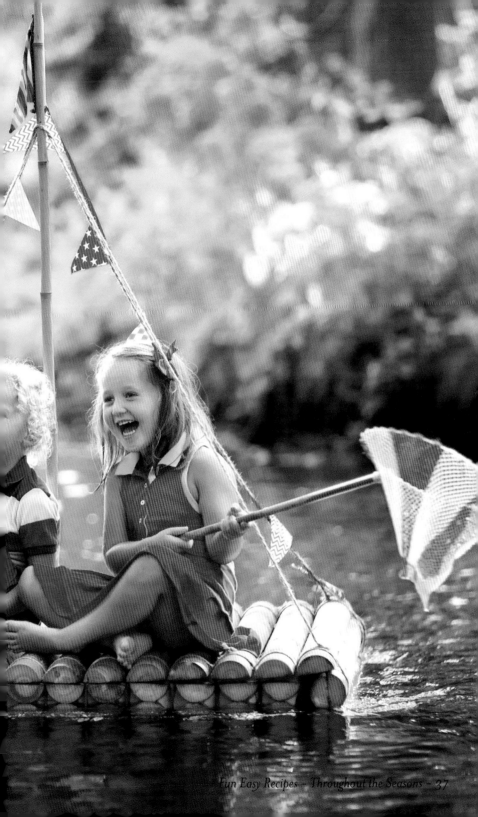

Summer Relaxation Body Scrub

Ingredients:
- 4 drops Lavender Essential Oil
- 4 drops Geranium Essential Oil
- ½ cup Raw Sugar
- ¼ cup Virgin Coconut Oil
- 4 oz Glass Mason Jar

Directions:
1. Put the Raw Sugar, Coconut Oil, Lavender and Geranium Essential Oils into a glass bowl
2. Mix the ingredients together
3. Place the mixture into the jar
4. Use this scrub to exfoliate and calm your body

Ocean Mist Air Freshener

Ingredients:
- 3 drops Citronella Essential Oil
- 3 drops Lemongrass Essential Oil
- 3 drops Spearmint Essential Oil
- 3 drops Orange Essential Oil
- Water
- 2 oz Glass Spray Bottle

Directions:
1. Add the Essential Oils into the spray bottle
2. Fill with water and put on the spray bottle top
3. Shake well before spraying into the air

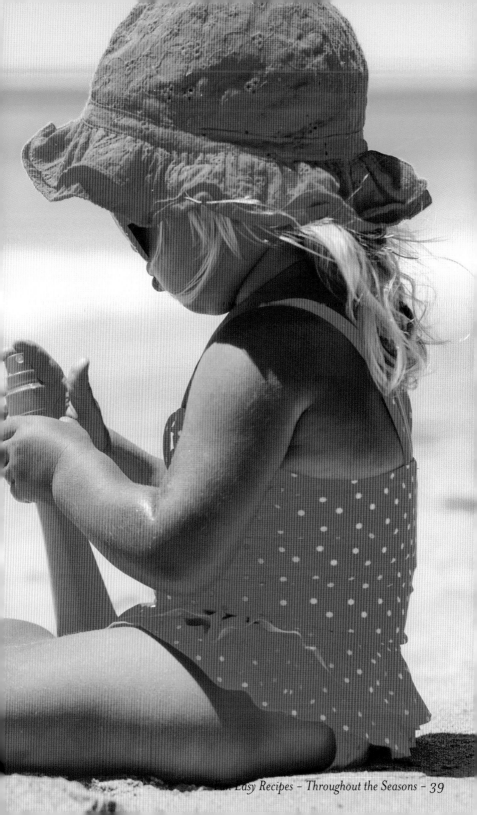

Citrus Loving Diffuser Blend

Ingredients:
- 2 drops Grapefruit Essential Oil
- 3 drops Citrus Fresh Essential Oil
- Water
- Diffuser

Directions:
1. Add water to the fill line of the diffuser
2. Put Grapefruit and Citrus Fresh Essential Oils into the water
3. Put the top of the diffuser on and press the on button
4. Breathe in the happiness of the citrus scents

Vacation Time Bath Salts

Ingredients:
- 3 drops Stress Away Essential Oil
- 3 drops Ylang Ylang Essential Oil
- 3 drops Lavender Essential Oil
- 1/3 cup Epsom Salt
- 4 oz Glass Mason Jar

Directions:
1. Put the Epsom Salt, Stress Away, Ylang Ylang and
   Lavender Essential Oils into a glass bowl
2. Mix the ingredients together and place the mixture into the jar
3. Add 1 tablespoon of the mixture into your bath
   water to create a vacation time experience

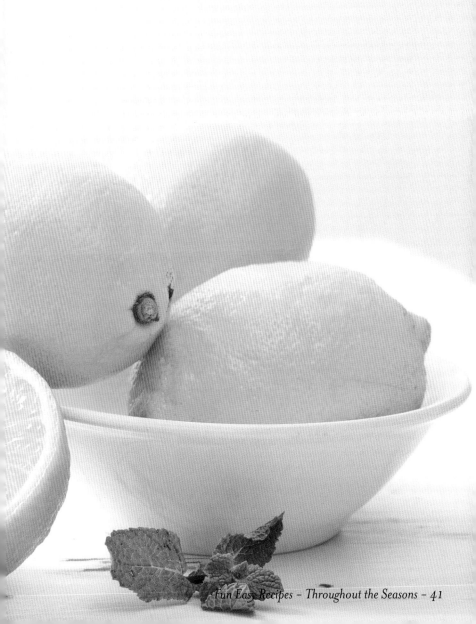

Grapefruit Lime Sugar Scrub

Ingredients:
- 4 drops Grapefruit Essential Oil
- 4 drops Lime Essential Oil
- ½ cup Raw Sugar
- ¼ cup Virgin Coconut Oil
- 4 oz Glass Mason Jar

Directions:
1. Put the Raw Sugar, Coconut Oil, Grapefruit and Lime Essential Oils into a glass bowl
2. Mix the ingredients together
3. Place the mixture into the jar
4. Use this scrub to exfoliate your hands or body, while uplifting your emotions

Summer Time Body Spray

Ingredients:
- 4 drops Ylang Ylang Essential Oil
- 4 drops Lavender Essential Oil
- Water
- 2 oz Glass Spray Bottle

Directions:
1. Add the Essential Oils into the spray bottle
2. Fill with water and put on the spray bottle top
3. Shake well before spraying onto your body

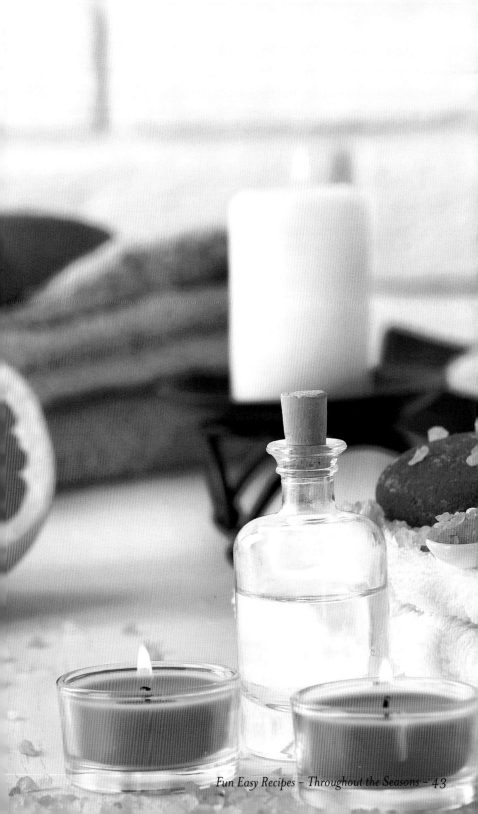

Summer Bliss Diffuser Blend

Ingredients:
- 3 drops Citronella Essential Oil
- 2 drops Lemongrass Essential Oil
- Water
- Diffuser

Directions:
1. Add water to the fill line of the diffuser
2. Put Citronella and Lemongrass Essential Oils into the water
3. Put the top of the diffuser on and press the on button
4. Breathe in the happy scents of Summer

Cooling Roll-On

Ingredients:
- 10 drops Peppermint Essential Oil
- V-6 Vegetable Oil (or Liquid Coconut Oil)
- 10 mL Glass Roll-On Bottle

Directions:
1. Add the Peppermint Essential Oil into the roll-on bottle
2. Fill with V-6 Vegetable Oil and put on the roll-on top
3. Apply onto the back of your neck

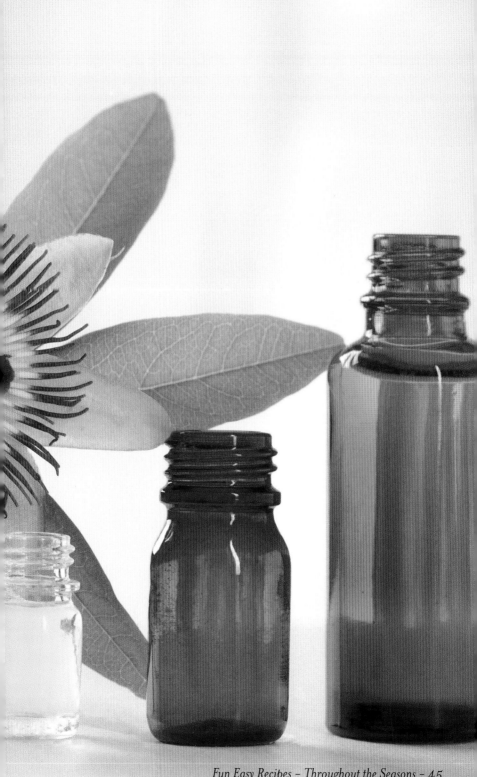

Soothing Skin Cream

Ingredients:
- 8 drops Lavender Essential Oil
- 2 drops Frankincense Essential Oil
- 1 Tbsp Aloe Vera Gel
- ¼ cup Virgin Coconut Oil
- 4 oz Glass Mason Jar

Directions:
1. Add the Lavender and Frankincense Essential Oils, Aloe Vera Gel and Coconut Oil into a glass bowl
2. Mix the ingredients together
3. Place the mixture into the jar and apply to skin when needed

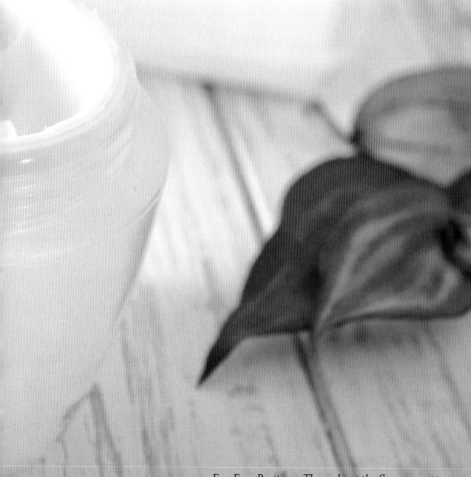

After Swimming Roll-On

Ingredients:
- 7 drops Ledum Essential Oil
- 5 drops Thieves Essential Oil
- V-6 Vegetable Oil (or Liquid Coconut Oil)
- 10 mL Glass Roll-On Bottle

Directions:
1. Add the Essential Oils into the roll-on bottle
2. Fill with V-6 Vegetable Oil and put on the roll-on top
3. Apply onto the bottom of the feet after swimming
   to support the immune system

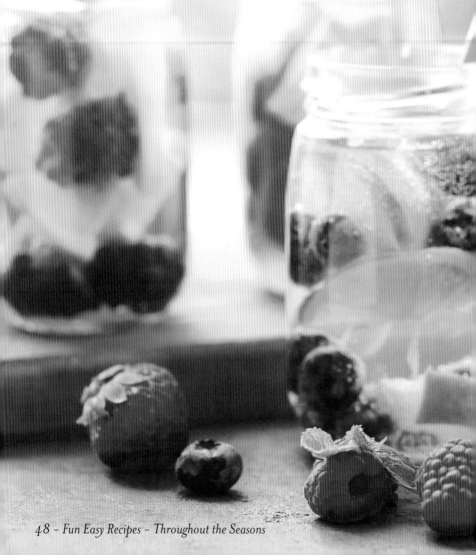

Strawberry Lemonade

Ingredients:
- 2 drops Lemon Vitality Essential Oil
- 12 oz Fresh Strawberries
- ½ gallon Organic Lemonade

Directions:
1. Place the strawberries and half of the lemonade into a blender, blend well
2. Pour mixture into a glass pitcher and add in the rest of the lemonade and Lemon Vitality Essential Oil
3. Mix well and enjoy .

Frozen Berry Lime Margarita

Ingredients:
- 2 drops Lime Vitality Essential Oil
- 1 lb Frozen Strawberries
- ½ cup Orange Juice
- 2 Tbsp Raw Sugar

Directions:
1. Add the strawberries, orange juice and raw sugar into a blender, blend well
2. Pour mixture into a glass pitcher and add the Lime Vitality Essential Oil
3. Mix well and enjoy

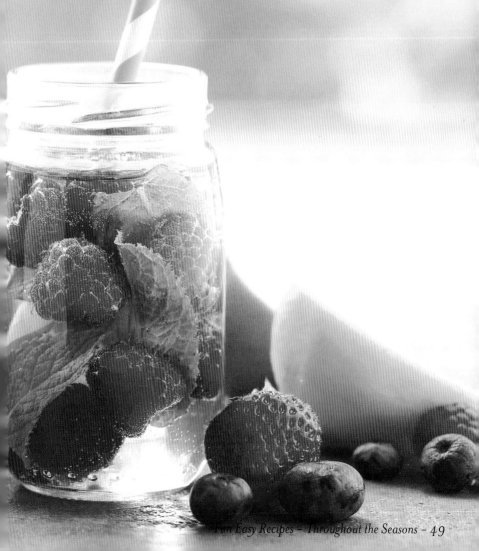

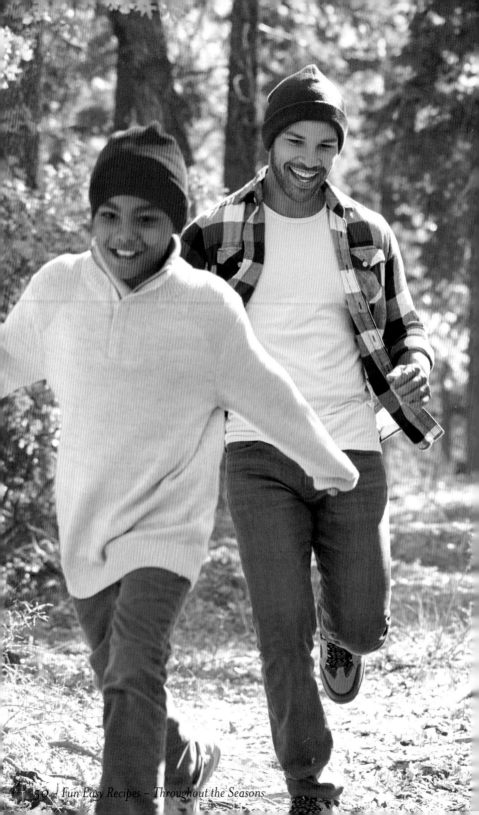

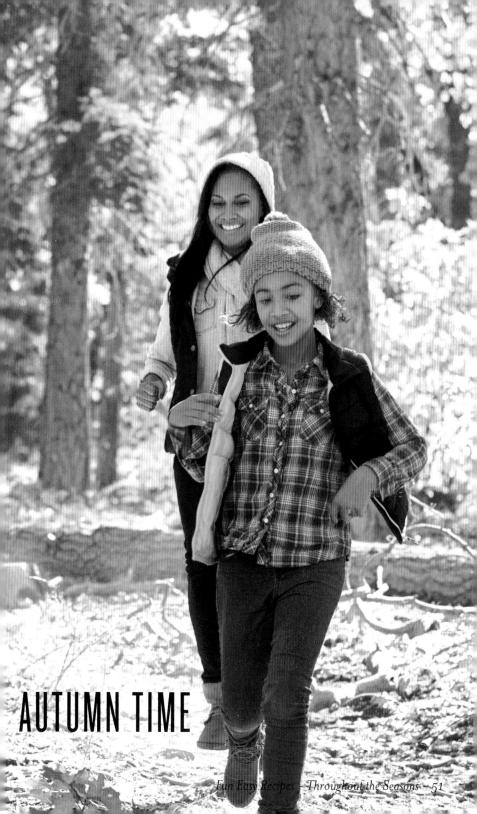

AUTUMN TIME

Autumn Breeze Roll-On

Ingredients:
- 6 drops Orange Essential Oil
- 4 drops Ginger Essential Oil
- 4 drops Thieves Essential Oil
- V-6 Vegetable Oil (or Liquid Coconut Oil)
- 10 mL Glass Roll-On Bottle

Directions:
1. Add the Essential Oils into the roll-on bottle
2. Fill with V-6 Vegetable Oil and put on the roll-on top
3. Apply onto your wrists as an Autumn perfume

Sugar & Spice Room Spray

Ingredients:
- 6 drops Cinnamon Bark Essential Oil
- 5 drops Nutmeg Essential Oil
- 5 drops Orange Essential Oil
- Water
- 2 oz Glass Spray Bottle

Directions:
1. Add the Essential Oils into the spray bottle
2. Fill with water and put on the spray bottle top
3. Shake well before spraying into the air

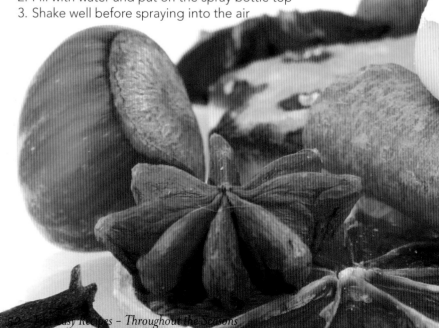

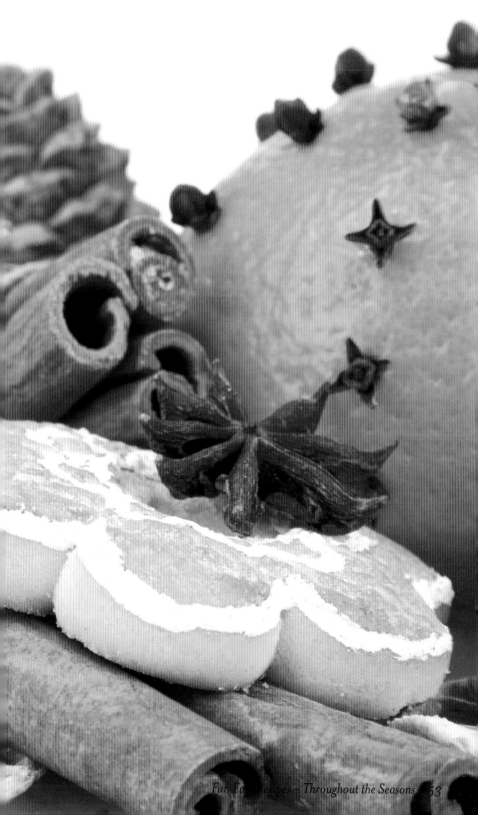

Autumn Time Sugar Scrub

Ingredients:
- 3 drops Clove Essential Oil
- ½ tsp Vanilla Extract
- ½ cup Raw Sugar
- ¼ cup Virgin Coconut Oil
- 4 oz Glass Mason Jar

Directions:
1. Put the Raw Sugar, Coconut Oil, Vanilla Extract and Clove Essential Oil into a glass bowl
2. Mix the ingredients together
3. Place the mixture into the jar
4. Use this scrub to exfoliate your hands or body

Yummy Apple Pie Diffuser Blend

Ingredients:
- 2 drops Cinnamon Bark Essential Oil
- 2 drops Ginger Essential Oil
- 2 drops Clove Essential Oil
- Water
- Diffuser

Directions:
1. Add water to the fill line of the diffuser
2. Put Cinnamon Bark, Ginger and Clove Essential Oils into the water
3. Put the top of the diffuser on and press the on button
4. Breathe in the yummy scent of apple pie

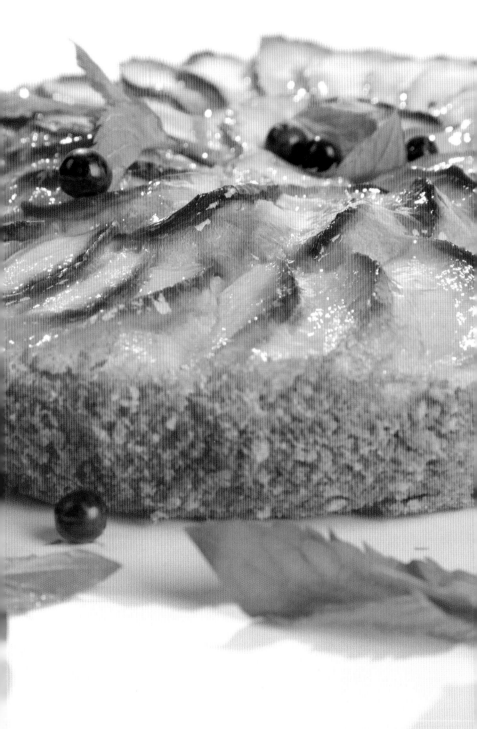

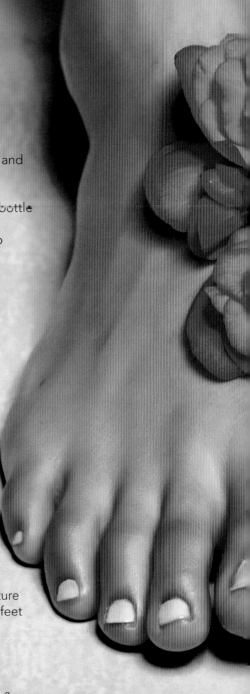

Pumpkin Spice Foaming Hand Soap

Ingredients:
- 4 drops Cinnamon Bark Essential Oil
- 4 drops Orange Essential Oil
- 4 drops Clove Essential Oil
- 3 Tbsp Castile Soap
- Water
- 8 ½ oz Glass Foaming Bottle

Directions:
1. Add Cinnamon Bark, Orange and Clove Essential Oils into the foaming bottle
2. Add Castile Soap and fill the bottle with water
3. Put on the foaming bottle top
4. Use this to wash your hands

Fall Delight Foot Soak

Ingredients:
- 3 drops Thieves Essential Oil
- 5 drops Orange Essential Oil
- ⅓ cup Epsom Salt
- 4 oz Glass Mason Jar

Directions:
1. Put the Epsom Salt, Thieves and Orange Essential Oils into a glass bowl
2. Mix the ingredients together and place the mixture into the jar
3. Add 1 tablespoon of the mixture into a foot bath to relax your feet

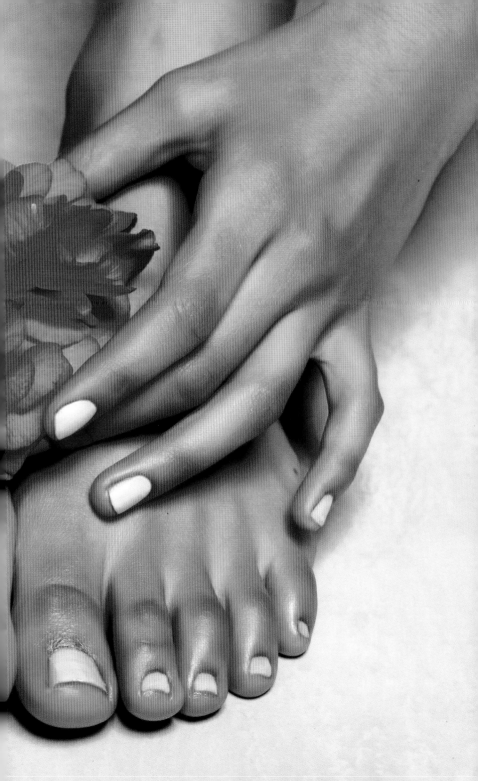

Autumn Spice Diffuser Blend

Ingredients:
- 2 drops Cinnamon Bark Essential Oil
- 2 drops Orange Essential Oil
- 2 drops Tangerine Essential Oil
- Water
- Diffuser

Directions:
1. Add water to the fill line of the diffuser
2. Put Cinnamon Bark, Orange and Tangerine Essential Oils into the water
3. Put the top of the diffuser on and press the on button
4. Breathe in the Autumn scents throughout your home

School Days Immune System Support

Ingredients:
- 10 drops Thieves Essential Oil
- 5 drops Frankincense Essential Oil
- 5 drops Thyme Essential Oil
- 5 drops Oregano Essential Oil
- V-6 Vegetable Oil (or Liquid Coconut Oil)
- 10 mL Glass Roll-On Bottle

Directions:
1. Add the Essential Oils into the roll-on bottle
2. Fill with V-6 Vegetable Oil and put on the roll-on top
3. Apply onto your children's spine and the bottom of their feet each day

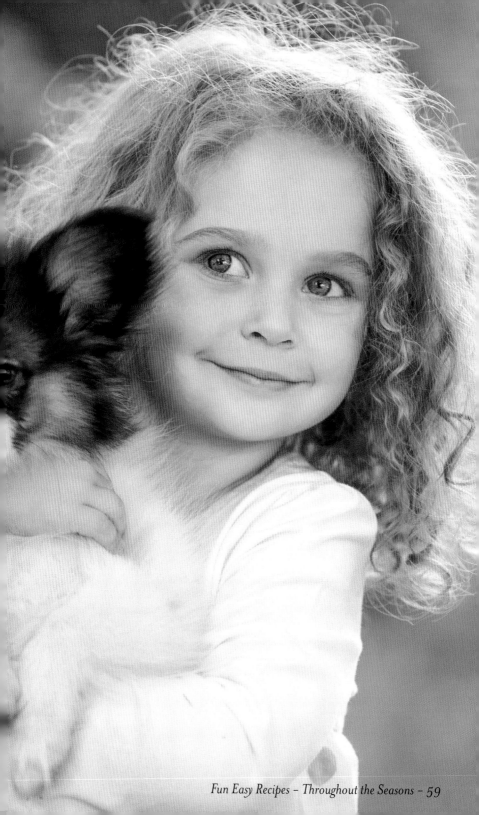

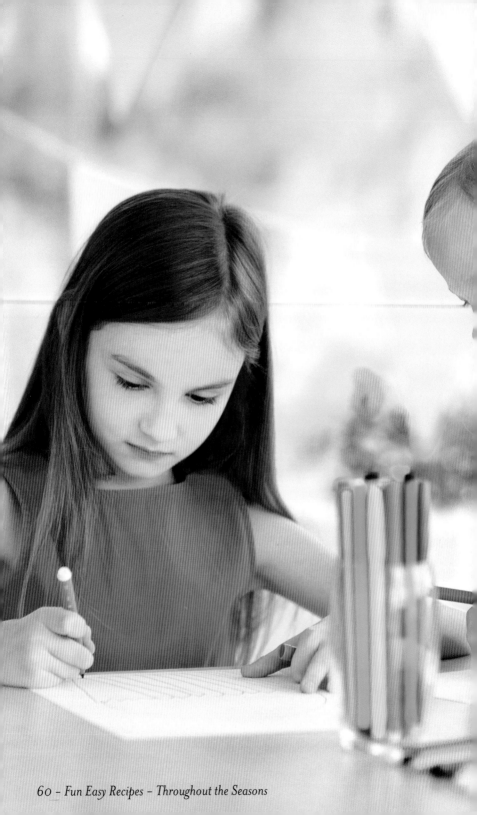

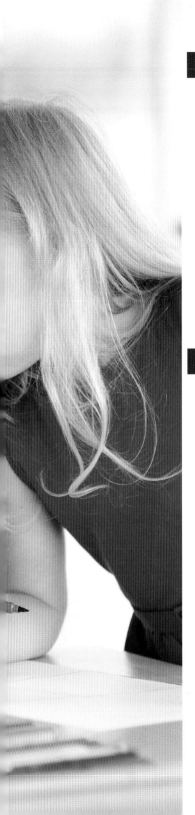

Healthy School Time Hair

Ingredients:
- 8 drops Lavender Essential Oil
- 8 drops Rosemary Essential Oil
- 8 drops Tea Tree Essential Oil
- Water
- 2 oz Glass Spray Bottle

Directions:
1. Add the Essential Oils into the spray bottle
2. Fill with water and put on the spray bottle top
3. Shake well before spraying into your children's hair

Homework Time Roll-On

Ingredients:
- 5 drops Lavender Essential Oil
- 5 drops Valor Essential Oil
- 5 drops Cedarwood Essential Oil
- 5 drops Vetiver Essential Oil
- V-6 Vegetable Oil (or Liquid Coconut Oil)
- 10 mL Glass Roll-On Bottle

Directions:
1. Add the Essential Oils into the roll-on bottle
2. Fill with V-6 Vegetable Oil and put on the roll-on top
3. Apply onto the back of the neck before homework time

Dreamy Chocolate Smoothie

Ingredients:
- 2 scoops Chocolate Pure Protein Complete
- 1 Tbsp Peanut Butter
- 8 oz water
- ½ cup ice
- 1 Banana

Directions:
1. Place the water, Chocolate Pure Protein Complete, peanut butter and ice into a blender
2. Add the banana into the blender
3. Blend, then pour into a glass, drink, and enjoy

Hot Cinnamon Spice Drink

Ingredients:
- 1 drop Cinnamon Bark Vitality Essential Oil
- 1 drop Nutmeg Vitality Essential Oil
- 1 Tbsp Raw Honey
- 1 cup Water

Directions:
1. Heat up water and pour into a mug
2. Add the Essential Oils and raw honey
3. Mix together and drink

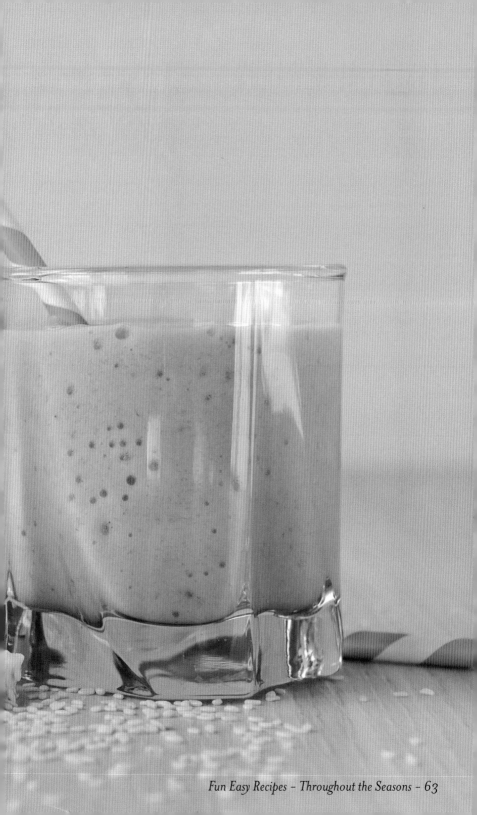

ESSENTIAL REWARDS

Save Money ~ Transfer Buy ~ Get Rewarded

- Receive 10-25% back in product credit EVERY MONTH and it's cumulative

- Redeem the points for FREE PRODUCTS!

- Receive Flat Rate and Reduced Shipping

- FREE GIFTS for members that stay on Essential Rewards for 3, 6, 9, and 12 months!

- Purchase your Healthy Lifestyle products through Young Living (ex: toothpaste, deodorant, shampoo, body wash, etc.)

- ONLY Requirement: place a 50 PV order each month

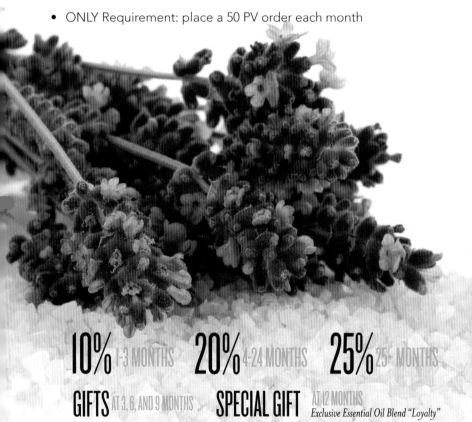

10% 1-3 MONTHS **20%** 4-24 MONTHS **25%** 25+ MONTHS

GIFTS AT 3, 6, AND 9 MONTHS   **SPECIAL GIFT** AT 12 MONTHS
Exclusive Essential Oil Blend "Loyalty"